Liver Cleanse Diet:

Natural Liver Cleansing Diet to Purify Your Liver, Detox Your Body and Increase Energy Levels

By

Brittany Samons

Table of Contents

Introduction 5

Chapter 1. Principles of a Liver Cleanse Diet 6

Chapter 2. How Can a Liver Cleanse Diet Help? 7

Chapter 3. Foods to Eat 11

Chapter 4. Foods to Avoid 14

Chapter 5. How to Use Liver Cleanse Diet Effectively? 15

Chapter 6. Sample Liver Cleansing Diet Plan 16

Chapter 7. Using Herbs and Natural Remedies 19

Chapter 8. Alternative Remedies for Liver Cleansing 23

Chapter 9. The Importance of Regular Liver Cleansing 25

Chapter 10. Using Liver Cleansing for Wellness 27

Thank You Page 28

Liver Cleanse Diet: Natural Liver Cleansing Diet to Purify Your Liver, Detox Your Body and Increase Energy Levels

By Brittany Samons

© Copyright 2014 Brittany Samons

Reproduction or translation of any part of this work beyond that permitted by section 107 or 108 of the 1976 United States Copyright Act without permission of the copyright owner is unlawful. Requests for permission or further information should be addressed to the author.

This publication is designed to provide accurate and authoritative information in regard to the subject matter covered. This work is sold with the understanding that the publisher is not engaged in rendering legal, accounting, or other professional services. If legal advice or other expert assistance is required, the services of a competent professional person should be sought.

First Published, 2014

Printed in the United States of America

Introduction

A liver cleanse is a cleansing diet that is meant to cleanse, detoxify and flush the toxins and dangerous microorganisms from the liver. The liver tends to become accumulated with toxins and dangerous chemicals that could cause illness, weakness and even cancer. Cleansing will help to reduce the symptoms that are associated with these conditions and will also prevent complications that could be a hindrance to optimum health and wellness.

The liver is an organ that acts like a strainer. It efficiently filters everything that the body takes in: food, medication, supplements, beverages and so on. It works 24 hours a day even when we are asleep or at rest. The liver works in conjunction with all other organs of the body to ensure that there is balance and efficient digestion and excretion of waste products in the body. When the liver is diseased, the body will accumulate toxins and dangerous chemicals in the blood which can lead to serious illness and complications.

Chapter 1. Principles of a Liver Cleanse Diet

Think of the liver as a sieve that traps all dangerous toxins and chemicals; it is important to remove all the trapped toxins from this sieve to ensure that the sieve is able to work efficiently once again. With a cleansing diet, the liver as well as all the organs that are related to digestion and excretion is cleansed. When a cleansing diet is meticulously followed there will be better function of these organs in the long run.

A cleansing diet is recommended at least once a month or once every two months to totally take advantage of the benefits of a liver cleanse. If you have never done a cleansing diet before then you will definitely feel different during the initial days of the diet. The reason for this is that there will be a stark change in your diet starting with some of your most favorite foods banned from your diet. It is also very hard to deal with a new diet especially when you find out the foods that are allowed and are not allowed in a liver cleanse diet.

Chapter 2. How Can a Liver Cleanse Diet Help?

A liver cleanse diet can help the body in so many different ways however it should be followed completely for the recommended number of days.

1. For better excretion of waste products – with a liver cleanse the liver is cleansed from toxins and other chemicals that can harm the kidneys and increase the risk of suffering from liver stones. Liver stones are made from accumulated minerals and toxins and these could impede the ability of the liver to filter the blood. Different sizes of stones with varying densities could develop and dislodge in the different structures of the liver and these could lead to inflammation, severe pain and a lot of complications. Although liver cleansing will not be effective in the removal of large liver stones it can help prevent the formation of new ones.

2. For better digestion- as mentioned, liver cleansing also involves cleansing other organs for digestion and excretion. Cleansing is like sweeping the colon from toxins, dangerous chemicals and microorganisms that can cause illness. You will be able to eliminate wastes regularly, avoid indigestion, prevent diarrhea and constipation, reduce bloating and gas formation. And when the body is able to digest various foods

efficiently there is also better nutrient absorption and calorie burn in foods that you eat.

3. For better cardiovascular health – better liver function benefits the entire body because blood that circulates the entire body is filtered efficiently. This reduces the risk of developing hypertension and increased cholesterol levels in the blood. You will also be able to reduce your chances of developing cardiovascular diseases and the risk of suffering from a stroke.

4. For healthier skin and hair – overall body health brought about by liver cleansing will also benefit hair and skin health. You will have stronger and healthier hair and scalp plus you will also reduce the symptoms of skin conditions like eczema and psoriasis.

5. For improved immunity – you will have overall improved immunity and this is evident as you have better control of your allergies, reduced incidence of upper respiratory infections like the common cold, cough, sore throat and so many more. You will also be in control of yeast or fungal infections that can lead to oral thrush, vaginal yeast infections, fungal infections of the skin and the colon.

6. For faster recovery from illness – when you have improved immunity you can be rest assured that you will easily recover from illness, infections and inflammation. You will experience faster wound healing time.

7. For prevention of illness, infection and cancers - with toxins removed from your body you will be able to prevent all sorts of illness, steer yourself from infection and there are also studies that prove toxins may cause cancers and efficiently removing toxins with a healthy and efficient liver will reduce the risk of suffering from cancers.

8. For prevention of premature aging – exposure to toxins from environmental pollution, chemicals from the foods that we eat and taking different medications exposes the body to harmful chemicals that can lead to premature aging. You can prevent signs of premature aging like poor skin health, poor eyesight, osteoporosis, poor memory and muscle weakness when you indulge in regular liver cleansing.

9. For weight loss – undoubtedly you will also experience weight loss when you do liver cleansing. As mentioned, liver cleansing is also in conjunction with colon cleansing wherein toxins, dangerous microorganisms and fat deposits are also removed from the body via the stool. This results in better absorption of nutrients from food to be utilized by the body

and of course better calorie burn which will gradually result to weight loss. When you indulge in regular colon and liver cleansing as well as eat a healthy diet and exercise you will be able to achieve weight loss and will also manage to keep the weight you lost off for good.

10. For improved psychological function and energy – liver and overall colon cleansing will benefit the entire body as well as the nervous system. You will eventually enjoy better concentration, better memory and increased reflexes. You will also have more energy to spare since you are able to digest foods better and absorb the nutrients from food as well.

Chapter 3. Foods to Eat

Just like any other diet the liver cleanse diet has a list of foods that are recommended for dieters. These foods will help facilitate cleansing and will help improve liver health.

Fiber-rich foods

You should eat more cruciferous vegetables like kales and cabbages, fruits like apples, pears, grapefruits, melons and papayas, leafy and green veggies and the usual vegetables like onions, cauliflowers and artichokes. These foods are rich in fiber which could add roughage in your stool. Fiber sweeps the colon clean by driving away toxins and dangerous microorganisms and excreting these via the stool.

Other fiber-rich foods that may also be used to improve colon and liver health are flax seeds, oats, brown rice and barley.

Protein rich foods

Proteins are important to build damage tissues and cells but you need protein sources that will not put a strain on the liver as it helps in digestion and filtering toxins. Therefore excellent protein sources may be found in dairy products, eggs, fish, seafood, soya beans and poultry.

Aside from these foods the body also needs foods that are great sources of nutrients like vitamins and minerals. These are usually found in fruits and vegetables as well as in legumes like lentils and kidney beans, various spices like cinnamon and garlic, seeds and nuts and so much more.

Organic foods

Eating organic foods is not a fad nor is it a hype. Organically-grown foods are fruits, veggies, meats and herbs that are grown and are cared for in the most natural manner. Fruits, veggies and herbs are grown in soils with low toxicity levels, without using herbicides, pesticides and fungicides while meats from farm animals like cows, chicken, goats, sheep and ducks are fed using organic materials and not chemically-processed feeds. You should search for a grocer or a market that sells organic foods or you may also grow plants and raise animals for food consumption on your own.

When it comes to fish, you should choose fish that are caught in the deep oceans where mercury and other toxic materials are at their lowest levels. You should be wary of shell fish like clams, mussels and oysters since there is a huge possibility that these are exposed to polluted sea water.

Drinking enough water each day

A crucial part of every cleansing diet is water. Water is a universal solvent and it reduces toxicity by diluting toxins and chemicals in the kidney as well as in the colon. It hydrates the body and keeps body temperature at the ideal level. Pure water is important so that the kidneys and the liver will never need to work hard in filtering the blood and urine. In every cleansing diet it is recommended that a dieter drinks as much as 10 or more glasses of water each day. Other types of liquids or beverage are prohibited especially commercially – prepared drinks, alcohol and drinks with caffeine.

Chapter 4. Foods to Avoid

It is important that anyone who wants to indulge in a liver cleanse diet to remember the foods that should be avoided. These foods are either processed, commercially-prepared or loaded with preservatives.

You should avoid commercially-processed meats, junk foods and preserved foods. Refined carbohydrates that are found in sweets, pastries, cakes, cookies and muffins should be avoided since these only contain ingredients that can harm the liver. Consuming a lot of alcoholic beverages should also be avoided since alcohol is damaging to the liver and kidneys. Finally taking supplements like nutritional supplements and liver-soluble vitamins should also be avoided since these will also overwork the liver. Any kind of food that will take time to digest will only overwork the liver and the gastrointestinal system and thus should be prohibited in a liver cleanse diet. Remember that the goal of live cleansing is to ease the work on the liver so that it would be able to heal and to return its efficiency in filtering blood.

Chapter 5. How to Use Liver Cleanse Diet Effectively?

There are different types of liver cleanse diet. Some diets require the dieter to follow a program that will take around 3 days while some may take 5 to 7 days a week. But all in all, if you wish to indulge in this diet plan you should commit at least a weekend as a part of this program. You need at least a Saturday or a Sunday so that you will be able to take a complete day's off. This diet plan may look easy but in the first few days you will feel weary and a bit anxious since you will be making a lot of changes in your diet. Resting is also a part of any cleansing program so that the body tissues and cells are able to recuperate.

Chapter 6. Sample Liver Cleansing Diet Plan

You need to create a liver cleansing diet diary to take note of the foods that you have eaten and any unusual symptoms that you may have felt as you indulged in the diet plan. A diary will also help in case you will indulge in this diet plan in the future.

1. As you indulge in a liver cleanse diet you should always eat light meals and light snacks. For breakfast you should eat cooked cereals, fruits and whole wheat bread. For lunch you should indulge in fish and poultry which should be preferably steamed or grilled. Fresh salads should be a part of every lunch and dinner meal and of course fresh fruits could replace sweet pastries and pies for dessert. For snacks, fruits, crunchy veggies and nuts.

2. Take a liver cleansing recipe. This is a recipe that has ingredients that will strengthen the liver and facilitates cleansing. This recipe needs Epsom salts about 3 tablespoons and about 3 cups of water. All you need to do is to mix the two ingredients together and then divide the mixture into four parts. Drink one part in the morning, the other one in the afternoon and the other one before you sleep. Reserve the fourth part of the mixture in the morning as soon as you

wake up. Refrigerate this mixture so you will be able to easily tolerate as you drink it. You may add maple syrup or honey to improve the taste of this mixture.

3. Prepare a mixture of half cup extra virgin olive oil and a cup of freshly-squeezed lemon juice. Ensure that this mixture is thoroughly mixed. You will drink this along with the Epsom salts mixture.

4. You use this liver cleanse recipe during the first day of your cleanse and repeat it during the final day regardless of how many days you are recommended to indulge on this diet plan.

There are other variations of a liver cleanse recipe like mixing lemons, flax oil, grapefruit, ginger root, garlic and live microorganisms like Acidophilus, mixing cranberry juice, cinnamon, nutmeg, ginger, lemon juice and flax seeds and a liver flush recipe consisting of citrus fruits, garlic, olive oil and ginger. If you have food allergies then you should consult your doctor or a dietician on the best ingredients that you may use for liver cleansing.

Drinking fruit and vegetable juices aside from water

As mentioned, pure water is preferred but you may also drink vegetable and fruit juices. You need to take advantage of the amazing fiber content of fruits and veggie so therefore you should drink your juices fresh.

A blender would be great in whipping up fresh fruits and vegetable juices but a more efficient way to use juice in cleansing is to use a juicer. There are different kinds and brands of juices but if you wish to juice up fruits with thick pulps and seeds then you should use a centrifugal juicer but if you wish to add herbs you should use a masticating type of juicer. You may juice up fruits in season like melons, berries, apples, pineapples, lemons and other citruses; for veggies you may juice up kales, cabbages, beets, carrots and ginger just to name a few. You may drink juice for breakfast and another glass of your choice for snacks of for diner.

Chapter 7. Using Herbs and Natural Remedies

Liver cleansing has been done in early times and in almost every culture, cleansing is done to purify the body from toxins and to reduce illness. Using an herb or a combination of herbs may be used as an effective liver cleansing formula.

1. Lemon juice – squeeze a medium sized lemon to get the juice and then dissolve this in a glass of lukewarm water; drink this at least once a day preferably before eating breakfast or before sleeping at night. Lemon has amazing natural properties that helps stimulate the liver to increase the production of bile. When the production of bile is increased toxins and chemicals are pushed out of the liver naturally. And as toxins are flushed from the body there will be a reduced risk in the development or buildup of stones in the liver. The gastrointestinal system also improves its ability to digest fats since the flow of gastric juices is also improved. Other variations of a lemon juice cleanse is drinking lemon tea. You can find preparer lemon teas in supermarkets or you may prepare your own by diluting two to three tablespoons of freshly squeezed lemon juice in a cup of warm water. You may add a teaspoon of maple syrup or honey to improve its taste.

2. Natural green tea – green tea is another way to flush out toxins from the liver and also helps improve liver health. Natural green tea is rich in antioxidants that can help boost the production of bile from the liver and just like lemon juice, can help flush out toxins since bile production is significantly improved. Fatty deposits from the liver are also removed while prevention of further accumulation of fatty deposits is reduced. Drinking green tea once in the morning during breakfast and once before sleeping at night is recommended. The ideal green tea is made from real green tea leaves and not commercially-prepared green tea products that you may find in convenience stores and supermarkets.

3. Eating foods rich in garlic is also a way to boost liver health. Make this as a part of your regular diet and not just during performing a liver cleanse. Garlic naturally has compounds that can stimulate enzymes that can flush out toxins from the body. The popular natural remedy also contains significant amounts of selenium and allicin which are important in liver health and detoxifying the liver and other organs for digestion. You may eat foods rich in garlic or you may take garlic supplements instead.

4. By eating fruits like avocadoes and grapefruit you can guarantee improved liver function and by combining it with a

liver cleanse, you will be able to reduce liver toxicity in no time at all. Avocadoes are known to have a high glutathione content; glutathione is a compound that can reduce liver toxicity by detoxifying the organ. Grapefruits on the other hand can boost a liver cleanse. It has natural compounds known as naringenin which can increase fatty deposit burn. These compounds also boost liver health.

5. Turmeric supplements are also known to help increase the success of a liver cleanse. This herb is known to have properties that can improve liver health and has been known to boost the regeneration of damaged liver cells. It is not surprising that you will find physicians recommending turmeric supplements to patients with fatty liver or liver disease like hepatitis. Take turmeric supplements as recommended by your doctor or according to package directions.

6. Using milk thistle is also a very popular liver cleansing strategy. Milk thistle is known to promote the regeneration of healthy liver cells. Milk thistle has natural compounds and silymarin that are powerful antioxidants that can stop cell oxidation of liver cells. Compounds that are also found in the liver may also improve protein synthesis and removal of fatty

deposits in the liver resulting in a healthy and fully-functioning organ.

Chapter 8. Alternative Remedies for Liver Cleansing

It is highly recommended that you also use alternative remedies to help boost liver cleansing. There are several ways to help jumpstart your cleansing even when you are at home.

1. Relaxation treatments are one of these alternative remedies and you can do this by the use of meditation, yoga or deep breathing exercises. If possible, perform relaxation activities in a quiet place in your house like a spare room or in a patio where you can take in fresh air. Listen to music or simply close your eyes so you can relax. These activities boost the body's ability to restore tissue function and health.

2. Engage in stress reduction activities. Being stressed will only affect your liver cleanse since you will never be able to engage in all the steps of the cleanse completely. Stress reduction may be done by engaging in hobbies, pastimes, sports, exercise activities and even by talking to someone about your stress. Having someone do liver cleanse with you is also known to improve compliance to the diet.

3. Reduce toxins and chemicals in your home. It's no use detoxifying the body when you are still surrounded by toxins. There are several ways to do it: you may use an air purifier at

home so you can clean air from allergens, toxins, dust and pollution; this is very important especially when you live in the city or near a roadway or where there is too much traffic. You should also consider using natural cleaning agents instead of using chemical cleaners. These cleaning agents are known to affect health and increases toxins in the air and in the home as well.

Chapter 9. The Importance of Regular Liver Cleansing

Liver cleansing should be done regularly and in fact all adults are recommended to engage in this diet at least once every two to three months to totally guarantee liver health. The liver works round the clock together with all the other organs of the body but it is the only organ that is affected by toxins the most. This is also very important to people that exposes themselves to toxins and chemicals. People that drink alcohol excessively (people with alcohol addiction), those that indulge in drugs, those with maintenance medication, those that take fad diets, those that take supplements without any regard to doctor's recommendation and so many more. All of these activities predisposes a person to overwork his liver and thus regular liver cleansing is a must. In regular cleansing, the following points should be remembered:

1. Cleansing should be done in a regular manner, do not skip or cheat. You are only cheating on yourself when you skip a day or decide to eat foods that are not allowed during the diet cleanse.

2. From now on you will avoid eating foods that should be avoided so that you will ease work on your liver. Alcohol

especially should be totally avoided. If you need help in stopping alcohol intake or taking care of alcohol addiction then you should seek help right away before indulging in a liver cleanse diet.

3. You should talk to your doctor about taking medications and supplements. Your doctor will help you find a more suitable way to take medications as you indulge in a liver cleanse diet.

4. Strive to stock up on veggies and fruits as well as all the other foods that are allowed in your diet. Overhaul your food stockpile and your refrigerator content so that you will less likely to relapse. You should also start thinking of growing your own veggies and herbs to ensure that you have a healthy supply of food items that are free from pesticides and chemicals.

5. Regular liver cleansing diets should be done only when you are feeling well enough. Do not try to use a liver cleanse diet when you are sick or you have gastrointestinal problems and liver damage. If you have a medical condition, talk to your doctor beforehand so you will know if you may indulge in a liver cleanse diet.

Chapter 10. Using Liver Cleansing for Wellness

Liver cleansing has been one of the oldest ways to bring good health. It is believed that the liver holds the key to good health and any illness is attributed to imbalances in the liver together with the other organs for digestion. These beliefs have been carried over till today and liver cleansing has been proven to totally improve the health and wellness of a person if the diet is carried out exactly as described.

A liver cleanse diet also promotes a whole body cleanse or a holistic cleanse simply because the liver is responsible for filtering the blood that runs through all the tissues, organs and body systems of the body. The blood supplies nutrients, sugar and oxygen in various tissues and organs and with a healthy blood a healthy body is eventually expected. Liver cleanse diets are also too good to keep on your own and therefore should be shared within your family and friends. This practice is very important since our friends and family greatly influences what we are and what we eat and consume as a beverage. You are more likely to stick to liver cleansing diets as a regular part of your life when other people are also doing the same thing.

Thank You Page

I want to personally thank you for reading my book. I hope you found information in this book useful and I would be very grateful if you could leave your honest review about this book. I certainly want to thank you in advance for doing this.

www.ingramcontent.com/pod-product-compliance
Lightning Source LLC
LaVergne TN
LVHW021748060526
838200LV00052B/3539